You Have An Ugly Baby

Nalin-
Thanks for your
friendship.

Don

You Have An Ugly Baby

The unpleasant truth about your
company's health care costs and how
you CAN change your destiny!

Daniel Rickard

2007

You Have An Ugly Baby

TABLE OF CONTENTS

To my wife, Floellen, whose relentless quest for the truth inspires me every day.

FOREWORD

First to those of you who I know, both friends and family, I'd like to say the title of this book has absolutely no reference to any of your children. I'd like to say that, but we both know that's not true. They are not all easy on the eyes.

Writing this book was easier than continuing to bite my tongue as health plans and their advisors continue to hurtle headlong in the wrong direction, sending companies and employees alike scurrying for financial shelter. It's simple, really: If your automobile insurance goes up because you have too many tickets or at-fault accidents, the answer is *not* a new car. The antidote is behavioral change, becoming a more responsible and conscientious driver.

Recently, several Fortune 500 companies have made headlines with VEBA Trusts and other creative financing strategies confusing cost shifting with cost control.

Centuries of persecution have dogged those who would proclaim obvious truths, like telling the emperor he has no clothes, and consequently silenced those bearers of unpleasant truths.

That is, until now.

RUNAWAY TRAIN

Debbie looked at her notes, at her watch, and then back at her notes. John, the CFO, was late, but it was just as well. She had no good answers, no solutions, nothing. Not one single solitary idea on how Goodman Products Co. could possibly mitigate the 15.8% increase projected for next year's health insurance cost.

Raise deductibles? Co-pays? Employee contributions? The 850 employees of Goodman had suffered through this "death by a thousand cuts" for the last several years. Cost shifting had left the building, but, frankly, the resulting employee noise had scarcely been worth the short-term relief.

Debbie truly loved being the director of human resources and the broad landscape of her responsibilities. The compliance issues were a pain but their nuisance was necessary, and she was a company first employee. Recruiting and training was always her first love and the reason she had pursued a degree in HR in the first place. Although she fully embraced the area of her studies dedicated to employee benefits, she never dreamed that managing the rising cost of health care would become the benchmark against which her career would be judged. It was a runaway train, and she was on it, too. Her ten-year-old daughter, Lauren, had been diagnosed with juvenile diabetes just two years ago, and Debbie struggled to stay objective when selecting which coverages to modify. Debbie's own financial burden connected her to the rest of Goodman's employees as they scrambled to pay 20% of their health care cost from an average company salary of just over $16 an hour.

The conference room phone interrupted her daydream and Debbie saw John Frank's number appear on the ID screen.

"Hi, John."

"Debbie, I'm sorry for keeping you, but I have to reschedule. Our auditors just showed up with last minute questions on our financials."

"No problem, John. I'll check your calendar and pull something together later this week."

"Thanks." Click.

Thank God for the auditors. Putting down the receiver, Debbie sighed, "Just as well."

As she walked down the long, gray hall toward her office, she couldn't help but remember her first interview at Goodman seven years earlier. Debbie recalled the pride she felt when she was offered the position and became the first degreed professional hired to fill the role of human resources director.

She felt her first order of business should be the basics: policies and procedures and the employee handbook. In an exercise that more resembled an archaeological dig, she finally located a three-ring binder stuffed with sticky notes, faxes on heat-sensitive paper, and yellowing copies of boilerplate documents from antiquated HR manuals yet to be completed. When the shock wore off, she dove in, and, in just three weeks, produced her first masterpiece, a true work of art consisting of a completely current policies and procedures manual that was not only compliant but available in electronic format as well.

The housekeeping that followed was more predictable: salary surveys, job descriptions, payroll interface (ugh), terminations, and team building with departmental managers. She even had time for the recruiting and training that had drawn her to human resources in the first place. Everything seemed manageable, solution-based, logically resolvable.

Everything was predictable except the health plan costs.

As Debbie sat down at her desk, she realized that this year was just like the year before, which was a carbon copy of the year before that. How, she wondered, could the wealthiest country in the world, with the brightest and best minds, not have a better solution to a problem so enormous that it was dragging companies of all sizes to financial ruin? Nothing seemed to change the outcome. Different insurance companies, networks, third-party administrators, and brokers all produced the same predictable result: higher costs.

Debbie leaned back and thought about the paper she wrote in her last year at college detailing the origin of health insurance.

It was 1929 when Dr. Justin Kimball left his job as a school superintendent to become the vice president at Baylor University in charge of the College of Medicine and the hospital. As he reviewed the list of overdue accounts, he recognized many of the names of Dallas schoolteachers he'd known from his previous work.

Knowing full well these low-paid educators would continue struggling to pay their bills, he created the "Baylor Plan," allowing teachers to pay fifty cents each month into a fund that guaranteed up to twenty-one days of hospital care at Baylor Hospital. As word spread to other hospitals across the country of the Baylor Plan, similar plans were set up. This led to the birth of modern health care as we know it. In 1944, the Baylor Plan became Blue Cross of Texas. Coverage for care provided by doctors was later added and was called Blue Shield.

It was a simple, functional idea. And now this "simple idea" had become the bane of Debbie's existence, a veritable minefield fraught with many moving parts, competing agendas, and a feeling of apathy from the general public.

Is it possible, she wondered, that the system is just too broken?

She shuddered to think of the alternatives: no health plan at all, social medicine that worked so well Canadians were stacked up at the border clamoring for treatment while OHIP (Ontario Health Insurance Plan) was barely financially treading water. In Europe, the United Kingdom's Tony Blair wrestled with the ethical ramifications of "QALYs," Quality Adjusted Life Years, essentially offering services only if outcomes balanced against costs. This, of course, was perfectly logical unless it was your eighty-year-old grandmother that needed a bypass. No single issue had fueled more incendiary debates between ethicists and economists.

Never mind the more global, far-reaching implications. In 2005, the latest available data showed the United States spent over two trillion dollars on health care, or $6,700 per person. That number represented 16% of the gross domestic product. That number was projected to be four trillion by 2015, representing over 20% of the GDP.

Health insurance expenses were now the fastest growing component for employers and, barring a dramatic change, would overtake profits by 2008. (McKinsey, September 2004)

It occurred to Debbie that in its simplest form, Goodman Products had neither a financial manager nor quality oversight for the single largest line item in the budget. This was not going to be pretty. She knew that premiums for employer-sponsored health insurance in the United States were rising four times faster than an average worker's salary.

Feeling the full weight of the health care budget debacle, Debbie knew it was time to change the game. Doing more of the same would inevitably produce more of the same dismal results that would bring Goodman one step closer to joining the ranks of 9% of companies eliminating health care from 2000 to 2005.

Her current broker had become nothing more than a delivery service, simply bringing in each year's bad news in the form of renewal increases with apologies and resignation. That had to change as well. Somewhere there had to be someone who felt the same sense of urgency that was consuming her at this moment. The weight grew heavier still when Debbie realized in her heart that it would likely fall to her to communicate the bad news to the executive team.

In that moment, she made a decision that would change everything she knew about benefits: she decided that the truth and only the truth would provide an opportunity to get off this runaway train.

She would have to tell the CEO the truth, "You have an ugly baby."

The implications could potentially be far reaching, but repeating failures of the past would surely be worse, especially when she had heard through the Goodman rumor mill that balancing the budget next year would simply be a function of health care cost increase = salaries eliminated. No one would be safe, including members of the executive team. Finding a solution now had the additional pressure of saving the jobs of those with whom she worked. She felt a little queasy inside knowing full well that the careers of many of her coworkers now depended on her ability to find a solution. It was also not lost on her that corporations tended to kill messengers without regard to the real root cause of the bad news.

As she stopped by the pharmacy for Lauren's insulin, she contemplated the outcome of her presentation to the executive team. It then occurred to her that her daughter's illness was part of the problem as well.

NEW DAY

The next morning, Debbie arrived earlier than usual with a renewed vigor and an excitement that surprised even her. She kicked out a quick e-mail to John, indicating that she needed a little more time to prepare for their benefits budget meeting.

John responded, "No problem." The auditors, Debbie mused, are now my new best friends.

She quickly located the last few years' benefit budgets and reviewed the changes. In the last few years, office visit co-pays had tripled along with deductibles. Prescription co-pays had similarly increased, prompting the company to offer a high-deductible plan with a Health Savings Account. This new wave product was touted as the next big thing, and John had insisted its inclusion at the eleventh hour despite Debbie's protest that lack of education would most certainly guarantee low participation. When only two employees enrolled (John was one), the air between them cooled considerably, and Debbie never had to say "I told you so."

Changes were also made that would affect her personally. Transplants were now the exclusive domain of "Centers of Excellence," which Debbie worried might preclude a provider that discovered a cure or treatment for Lauren's diabetes. A pancreatic transplant lay down the road if a cure could not be found, and the thought of having providers mandated smacked of the early days of HMOs.

Last year's changes had included disease management, which at first blush seemed to make sense. The problem was, of the eighty-six employees who had been identified as having one or more risk factors (her new word last year was "co-morbidity," which she learned was the combination of two or more risk factors like hypertension and elevated cholesterol), only three had actively engaged the resources provided by the disease management program. Clearly, there was a disconnect between those identified and their corresponding desire to manage or improve their health.

In the midst of all the paperwork, Debbie came across a hand-written note she recognized from her research last year. Although somewhat initially offended by the quote she had gleaned from the web, she nevertheless wrote it down: *"Americans want the best health care someone else's money can buy."*

Ouch!

She also came across an article clipped from one of the many journals that came across her desk regarding special drugs and their 28% rate of inflation. Clearly a fourth Rx co-pay tier should have been considered last year, but Debbie hadn't pushed. Lauren's chance for normalcy could someday appear and be classified in this specialty category.

"If the fire marshal catches you with that mountain of paper, you may be charged with arson!"

Debbie looked up to see Brenda, a member of her HR team, standing in the doorway.

"Whatever you're working on will probably look better on a full stomach. Let's grab some lunch, I'm starving," Brenda said.

Debbie wanted to continue, but thought that Brenda's fresh eyes might provide valuable insight. "Alright, let's go." "Walking or driving?" Debbie queried looking for her keys.

"Walking, I need the exercise, Deb."

Debbie locked her file cabinet, cursed HIPAA under her breath, and was out the door with Brenda.

"Brenda," she began between forkfuls of her chicken Caesar salad, "what do you think we should do about controlling our rising health costs? I'm concerned that we may lose good people if we can't balance the benefit budget."

"Well, for starters, I don't think you can control the costs, but I do believe they can be managed," said Brenda.

Debbie thought about Brenda's words then said, "I'm listening."

"Do you remember that seminar you sent me to last year? The one put on by that benefit consultant? Well, they talked about the disconnect between employee behavior and consequence, as well as the failure to use proper criteria in the selection process for vendors. I think I still have my notes if you want to see them."

Intrigued, Debbie sat up. "I'd like to see them, but I also want to know what you think. Did you get the feeling that there might be an answer or two in that seminar?"

Brenda crumpled her napkin into her plate and continued, "They talked about a lot, sort of a general indictment of everyone in the industry. What stuck in my mind were things like eighty-seven cents of every dollar spent on health care is a claim dollar, so why are you focusing so much time and energy on the fixed cost? They also stressed the fact that quality matters. They cited the results from a study—I believe it was from Dartmouth University—essentially equating higher quality of care with lower costs. It made sense at the time, but we were so busy slicing and dicing deductibles and co-pays, you know, that I got sidetracked and filed my notes away. I guess the statistic that bothered me the most was the reference to hospital quality."

"What about it?" asked Debbie, now thoroughly intrigued.

Brenda looked up as if to read it from a blackboard on the ceiling. "I believe the quote was 'If ninety-five percent of the hospitals performed at the quality level of the top five percent in several categories, over 50,000 deaths could avoided.' That just seemed tragic to me."

As they left the restaurant, Debbie asked Brenda again, "Do you think there's something there, I mean, did it strike you that what you heard might have application to our company?"

Brenda nodded her head up and down. "It won't be easy, but if you're willing to change the way you think about benefits, I think they're on to something. It was so simple, I didn't give it the credit it deserves, but it obviously stayed with me."

Debbie's pace picked up as they walked back to the office. "Brenda, I want you to get someone from any department other than HR to work with you and me on this project. Our time table is compressed, but it sounds like your notes may be the key to managing our health care cost *and* saving jobs."

"I know right where they are," said Brenda, "and I know exactly who to recruit for our team!"

Debbie allowed herself the first smile since yesterday's cancelled meeting with John. Maybe, she thought, there's a way out after all.

HOW DID WE GET HERE?

With the DND button activated on her phone, Debbie blocked most of the next day and poured over the notes Brenda had taken a year earlier. Some of the ideas seemed vaguely familiar, but others she was clearly seeing for the first time. Included in Brenda's notes was a timeline that resembled this:

- 1929—Health care invented
- 1981—Traditional health plans
- 1988—HMO
- 1991—Point of Service
- 1994—PPO
- 2001-CDH-HRA/HSA

As Debbie reviewed the progression and resulting plan designs, something jumped out at her. The traditional plans offered years ago had high deductibles and no prescription coverage, bearing a striking resemblance to the "Consumer Driven, High Deductible" health care plans she had implemented last year.

"How ironic," she said to no one in particular. "Thirty years later and we're right back where we started."

She reviewed the information detailing the competing agendas of the HMO structures, learning about capitation and the responsibility of gatekeepers. HMOs had their share of functionality issues, but the underlying theme of "Maintaining Health" was essentially on target. They just went about it the wrong way and in the process contributed their fair share to rising costs.

For instance, removing the cost barrier to office visits by charging office visit co-pays certainly made it easier and more affordable to see your family physician. The theory was that encouraging people to seek care more often resulted in better overall health.

What happened in actual practice, of course, was far different. People covered by HMOs stopped thinking about whether or not a physician's attention was actually necessary and with no financial barrier sought care for every little thing.

Debbie remembered the home remedies in her childhood of "feed a cold, starve a fever" or was it the other way around? She thought back to the time she cut her arm on a wire fence, about her father applying butterfly bandages to close the wound and that horrible orange substance spread over the top to prevent infection. That same accident today would require the patient be rushed to the emergency room, seen by a triage nurse, then a doctor, with another one of them determining whether or not a plastic surgeon should be called in.

Point of Service plans, as they were called, recognized the possibility that not all necessary care was available inside the HMO network of providers. POS plans provided the option to seek care outside the network, while providing that, if so chosen, patient cost would be higher than care sought inside the HMO network. Each time service or care was necessary, the patient would have the choice of care either in the HMO or outside the HMO network, at the *Point of Service*.

Preferred Provider organizations, or PPOs, offered a wider range of providers without leaving the network, although the premise was still based on savings realized when services rendered were billed at previously negotiated prices consistent with joining the network. Providers within all of these networks benefited from an increase in patients as lower out-of-pocket costs steered patients into their facilities.

The first Rx card was also a new addition to the afore mentioned plan designs and replaced satisfying deductibles with flat dollar copays. This structure, with deductibles too, was ironically being resurrected as companies struggled to curb their health care cost escalation. Deductibles started appearing in pharmacy benefits four years ago.

Among the historical perspectives, Debbie saw numerous references alluding to the possibility of government health or social medicine. She took a deep breath and tried to visualize the outcome. Government health care brought to you fresh from the organization that brought you the $200 hammer and the $5,000 toilet seat.

While she was the first to admit that something was wrong with a system where 47 million people were uninsured, she doubted that the government's layers of bureaucracy would provide health delivery in a more affordable or more efficient fashion. In fact, of everything she now knew and believed to be true, government intervention would be a disaster of epic proportion. In fact, the government did have two health plans currently in operation. Medicare was on the verge of bankruptcy and Medicaid was rife with fraud.

Debbie thought back to the history of benefits at Goodman. When she arrived, Goodman Products offered a couple of PPO options which were self-funded and a fully insured HMO. Employee contributions were almost equal for all plans, so virtually all employees were in the richest PPO plan. Because the HMO was the least expensive, most of the younger, healthier employees chose this option. It seemed like a well thought out offering, and employees were generally happy.

Problem was, nobody ever stopped to think about the financial implications. In a fully insured plan like the HMO, the company paid a premium and the money was then gone, whether or not a claim was ever paid. In a self-funded program, the company hired a claims payer, called a third-party administrator, who paid the employees' medical claims in lieu of a premium.

When both plans were offered, healthier, younger people who did not plan on accessing medical care chose the less expensive HMO, while older, less healthy employees chose rich plans that paid medical bills at higher rates and allowed them to access care across a broader landscape of providers.

In one of her continuing education classes, Debbie learned about the phrase *"selecting against yourself,"* which was exactly what was happening at Goodman. Amid much grumbling, her first major change was to eliminate the HMO plan, which she had considered a dinosaur anyway. The result was the migration of the healthier population into one of the self-funded plans to get the advantage of their lower claims cost, which was less than the insured premium paid to the HMO.

Robert, the benefits consultant, had sort of come along with the job. He was likeable, somewhat attentive, and tried to be helpful. Robert made efforts at marketing the plans each year, but the results never delivered any earth shattering news. John, the company's CFO, found it difficult to get excited about saving $8,100 on the life plan when the increase on the company's $6 million health care tab was over one million dollars.

Robert's primary strategy to help mitigate the company's increases could be summed up in two words: Cost Shift.

Employees had a valid reason for being apprehensive at open enrollment time. Goodman Products had a great track record of reinforcing this apprehension as the company systematically neutralized recent pay raises with increases in the employee contributions for health care. The erosion in take home pay was staggering, and not just at Goodman Products, either, with American workers paying an average of 143% more for coverage today than in 2000, while their out-of-pocket costs for deductibles and co-pays rose 115% during the same period. (Hewitt Associates Nov 2004)

In reality, Robert was probably no different than the myriad of brokers who called on Debbie with some degree of regularity. He meant well, but had become entrenched in a standardized, time honored tradition of RFPs and business as usual. They all promised "great service" and the utilization of technology to identify claim drivers. But as she poured through the benefits history of Goodman Products, one thing became clear: *You can't run from your claims!*

Debbie also knew full well that the odyssey from one carrier to another had been futile. The drill was essentially the same. Robert would gather the data and send it out to the usual suspects, who would in turn underwrite to come up with their best guess as to the company's risk or claims exposure for the ensuing year. Then there would be the inevitable haggling when purchasing got involved trying to negotiate lower rates with no real reason or logic supporting the demand for lower premiums or rates. Finally, the insurance carrier who was currently best positioned to "buy" the company's business would step up, the change would be made, and Goodman Products was off to the races.

That was until the next year, of course, when the company's claims experience exposed the under-priced bid from the previous year which, of course, now needed to be balanced with a hefty rate increase. This process not only had a predictable outcome, it was extremely time intensive and created a myriad of issues for employees who were forced to constantly change providers when new carriers and networks came into play. Needless to say, Debbie was not looking forward to another "go to market" experience.

From the carrier side, another trend was developing as well. Goodman had changed carriers three times in the last five years, and now those carriers had a less than stellar opinion about any potential loyalty or partnership with the company. This in turn reduced their inclination to get very competitive for business they knew would be heading out the back door next year.

Debbie then came across a newspaper headline that ran a chill down her spine: *The uninsured population in the United States grew by 2.2 million to 47 million.* Debbie's challenge was to keep Goodman's employees off that list.

INSIDE THE NUMBERS

Far from being a mathematical equation to be solved numerically, the numbers provided insight, illuminating the true nature of trend and cultural predisposition toward fast food and low activity.

Debbie thought back to a recent movie "Super Size Me," in which Morgan Spurlock's thirty-day journey through a fast food menu transformed an otherwise lean, healthy individual into an obese, sickly, emerging high-risk patient. His point was dramatic and poignant: We are truly what we eat. Obesity had now passed smoking as the number one driver of health claims and showed no signs of slowing down. Ironically, the expansive growth of the fast food industry as well as the video game culture appeared to parallel or possibly be a contributing factor in the recent rise in obesity. Coincidence?

The related claim cost, Debbie knew, was significant: $200 more per year for those who were obese vs. the rest of the population. Obesity was now a national epidemic, with the number of clinically obese children doubling in the United States in the last twenty years.

Debbie pondered the statistical data in Brenda's notes, thinking, "This future generation of pre-diabetics is going to crush their employers' health plans under the weight of claims necessitated by their lack of control today."

The United States today, she read on, currently spent in excess of $5,000 each year on health care for every man, woman, and child whether insured or not. That was a total of $2 trillion, or enough to qualify as the number one spender in the world.

Then Debbie read the bad news: When it came to quality, including outcomes, the United States was not even in the top twenty. In fact its global ranking in spite of its spending was a miserable thirty-first. She was shocked to learn that countries like Colombia and Morocco ranked higher than the United States. ("The World Health Report 2000")

What some would describe as the basic tenets of the country's democracy, free market economics, and the right to pursue legal remedy, were also major conspirators in this "coup de cost."

The subject of tort reform reared its head from time to time, Debbie knew, but was usually decried by the public at large, who demanded the right to be justly compensated(read lottery)when, in fact, a jury determined that medical culpability existed. This, in turn, drove medical malpractice insurance rates up; for example, rates were running about $277,000 for an OB-GYN in Michigan with no claims and a flawless record.

As with any proper business model, that cost of doing business was priced into the cost of services delivered and billed, and voila! Debbie sighed as she realized that she had just learned of yet another cost driver in the health plan.

The United States' free market economy also supported research and development in the pharmaceutical arena, providing an amazing array of miracle cures—but at a price few could afford. Pharmaceutical trends now easily outstripped the rate of inflation for other medical claims. Exponential advances in research and consumer demand for higher quality of life (in a pill form, of course) had merged to form the perfect storm of runaway inflation. Prescriptions as a class were clipping along at an inflationary rate of 7% annually, but that was misleading. *Specialty drugs* as sub-classes were now approaching 14% of the total spend with an inflation rate of 21%, and even though they now represented but a small percentage of scripts written, specialty drugs will represent 25% of the total drug spend in four years. (Express Scripts 2006 Trend Report) Included in this class of drugs were hypnotics (sleep aids), non-AIDS antivirus, stimulants (weight loss), and arthritis, MS, cancer, and anemia medication.

Debbie knew that there was no better example of the ethical dilemmas facing employers today than the vaccine providing protection against the Human papilloma virus, or HPV. All agreed on its merits and benefits; in fact, no one in his or her right mind could possibly argue otherwise. But the question became "who should pay the $500 for the injection?" Was the employer responsible? The employee? Debbie wondered aloud, "What truly is the moral ethical obligation to the workforce at large and where does personal accountability begin?"

At a time when costs were out of control and trending steeper yet, new opportunities to spend health care dollars were not at the top of any employer's wish list.

The recent upheaval over Canadian drugs and their import into the United States positioned U.S. pharmaceutical companies in an unwanted spotlight and again raised the question of whether it was appropriate to have free market agendas trumping access and affordability in health care.

That being said, Canada was facing its own crisis, from trying to balance OHIP's (Ontario Health Insurance Plan) rising trend in health-care claim liability with the exodus of Canadian-educated physicians chasing bigger dollars south of the border.

Over the last several years, advances in medical science had also positively impacted mortality, creating a society that, while living longer, also provided more years of pumping health care dollars into the system during those last additional high morbidity years.

As fate would have it, the United States had risen to the challenge. By eliminating physical education in schools and increasing access to higher calorie foods, the country had managed to stabilize the rise in life expectancy and this year even take it down a notch.

Other numbers popped up as Debbie continued her review of Brenda's notes and handouts. One recurrent theme was consistently clear: there was plenty of blame to go around, and none of the moving parts explored thus far was free from culpability.

When the Federal Accounting Standards Board decided to enforce section 106 requiring companies to immediately recognize the current and future cost associated with maintaining and administrating retiree medical plans as a current liability, it undermined the most pristine balance sheet casting a pallor over those organizations that provide such coverage. General Motors' FASB 106 liability, for example, was in excess of its current book value. On the heels of FASB 106 came GASB 45, the governmental/municipality version of this draconian law. These OPEBs (other postretirement employee benefits as they were now referred to) added yet another layer of cost to an already struggling behemoth.

A recent report from Moody's Investors Service showed that companies might get an added boost—beyond just a balance-sheet improvement—by transferring retiree heath care benefits to workers. The move could have a modest brightening effect on companies' corporate credit metrics.

The aforementioned increase in uninsureds provided the balance of the grist necessary for the political mill to continue its grind toward some form of socialized medicine. Uninsured was a relative and misunderstood term, Debbie learned. Turned out the United States had a bastardized form of social medicine in place today in various forms: Medicare provided substantial health care for those sixty-five and older, while Medicaid was designed as a state-delivered program available to those below a certain income level.

Debbie also knew from conversations with her neighbor, who worked at the local hospital, that hospitals knowingly took in people without insurance coverage and absorbed the cost of their treatment into the total costs for services and then rolled those costs up among those who did have insurance.

In the final analysis, the average employer will pay 13% more this year than last—or a staggering $7,700 per employee annually. The cost of health care is rising at 250% the rate of the GDP, so that a worker making $36,000 today will make $52,000 in ten years at today's rate of 4% inflation. Unfortunately, the cost of health care is currently rising at 10%-plus, meaning that the worker making $52,000 in ten years will pay $26,000 for health care.

Can somebody say "Stop the bus, I want to get off!"?

THE USUAL SUSPECTS

Absent a single, guilt-ridden suspect trapped under the weight of insurmountable damning evidence, Debbie's investigation fell victim to scope creep, revealing a wide array of co-conspirators.

The *third party payer system* ranked at the top of every politician's hit list when it was time to play the blame game at election time. The irony was that these same politicos shamelessly accepted a large portion of their campaign funds from the same corporations that they openly criticized.

Third party, Debbie knew, referred to the platform where one party sought medical services from a second party, the bills were paid by a third party (an insurance carrier or TPA), and the final financial obligation usually rolled up to the employer. Although under constant criticism, the much maligned insurance industry continued to function and, in most cases, thrived as a financially viable alternative continuing to elude it's harshest critics. And there was perhaps an unreasonable expectation here as well, based on this fact alone: The health care system existed to provide for *its stakeholders.*

Clearly, thought Debbie, those seeking care were not stakeholders. Publicly traded health insurance companies had the simple deliverable of providing shareholder value, and they accomplished this by charging a fair market price for services provided. Underwriting or evaluation of risk was a critical component of adequate profitable pricing.

One needed look no further than the impending collapse/consolidation of community-based, community-rated HMOs now utilizing life support themselves or becoming targets of acquisition due to financial failure. Adverse selection was leaving them with inadequate premiums to cover the claims of those in poor health.

Some pointed to this as a futuristic manifestation of the health care system in general without a massive overhaul.

Community rating, or the "Statue of Liberty Plan" (give us your tired, your weary, your chronically ill, and emerging high risk), placed equal financial burden on both the healthy and unhealthy. Insurance carriers who chose to "underwrite" or evaluate medical information prior to providing pricing, enticed healthy organizations with lower rates. When those organizations bolted for the shelter of lower rates, those left in the Statue of Liberty (hereinafter referred to as the SOL plan) now shared the company of other organizations like themselves whose demographics or negative claims experience became the proverbial millstone around their collective necks without an influx of healthy populations to help provide safety or ballast in the law of large numbers.

Adverse selection then became the exponential undoing of local community-rated plans and many others like them around the country.

Experience rating placed the risk on the insurance carrier, albeit on a modified basis. Underwriters actuarially estimated the total expected claim liability of a given employee population based on previous years claims experience, demographics, and plan design. Subsequent years included pricing adjustments reflective of current claims experience and changes to demographics and/or plan designs. Unlike the stock market, past performance in health care analytics was usually a pretty good indicator of future performance, although this had been one number that seemed to move in only one direction.

ERISA statues enacted in 1974 allowed employers to provide health care on a self-funded basis. Third-party administrators acted as claim payers utilizing employer funds to pay providers treating employees and their families. This was a new opportunity for transparency, allowing employers to operate on a pure play basis.

The key components for an effective self-funded arrangement are:

1. Provider Networks—A group of local or even national providers who agree to a discounted fee schedule or reimbursement rate when treating subscribers to their network. Think of it as paying wholesale in lieu of retail.

2. Insurance Companies—There's seemingly just no way to exclude them, although in this case their role is greatly diminished as providers of stop loss insurance or reinsurance. Still, this is an important piece of any plan to ensure that no one claim or particularly bad year threatens the financial integrity of the plan itself. Insurance carriers, true to their self-serving nature, also invented "lasering," the practice of excluding certain high cost claimants in ensuing years or placing a separate higher deductible.

Leveraged trend is the phenomenon that describes the impact inflation has on the cost of stop loss insurance. The same catastrophic loss today will cost 10% more next year thanks to inflation, and because the loss exceeds the stop loss threshold in both years, the insurance carrier assumes more risk with each passing year. Result: stop loss premiums increase even if your catastrophic losses don't. (You didn't think the insurance company was going to just eat that, did you?)

3. Pharmacy Benefit Manager—This company is responsible for monitoring and measuring the delivery of prescription drugs at a discounted price. There is also the presumption of

a sharing or pass through of the rebates so generously offered through the pharmaceutical companies themselves.

4. Network discounts are a great way to access medical care at wholesale prices. Problem is, what discount are you getting and on what starting price is the discount based? Some networks, including some of the larger nationwide networks, actually provide discounts and keep a portion of the very discounts they provide. Huh?

5. Third-party administrators (TPAs) originally performed a simple task: the bill for services came in and a check for payment was issued. Seems like pretty simple stuff. But that was then, this is now. Today's claims are underpinned by an intricate web of eligibility, redundancy, fraud, and alternative responsibility, to name just a few. Today's TPA must be armed with big time technology to provide the filters necessary to weed out 3%-6% of the cost/waste that comes through the claims system for payment. In Goodman's plan, that difference could be $250,000 or more.

The self-funded process then was an exercise in unbundling the package products offered by insurers and reconstructing the best in breed offered by each vendor. Companies found their cost was now truly reflective of their own experience and, more important, a snapshot of the health of their workforce.

Self-funding then was the most transparent method of providing health care—what you see is what you get. Well, sort of.

As she reviewed the different rating methodologies, there was one shadow looming that Debbie knew would not go away: medical trend. Its diabolical thread wove through every plan, every company, and had averaged over 8% annually over the last forty years regardless of financing mechanism. In the end, it was the single biggest factor.

Medical inflation, or trend, also meant that just freezing claims at current levels was a guarantee of increased cost next year. Regardless of the financing mechanism, the amount being financed was increasing year after year. All things being equal, this year's $5 million expenditure would likely eclipse $5.6 million next year, and so on. And this, as John had clearly communicated to Debbie, was unacceptable. Period.

If merely holding claims flat was an unacceptable outcome, then logic dictated a reduction in claims. And fewer claims could only be the result of healthier choices and a resulting healthier workforce.

And that's when the light came on.

WELLNESS
A ROSE BY ANY OTHER NAME…

The word wellness conjures a variety of images for everyone who has ever entertained the notion of the buzz word now heard 'round the health care world. Even the Department of Healthcare and Human Services has gotten into the act, declaring that "Seventy percent of all health issues are the direct result of behavior and or lifestyle."

There are fund-raising walks for this disease and runs for that one. Debbie's favorite was National Smoke Out Day, essential allowing those who didn't smoke to express their superiority by banding together once a year to shake their collective fingers at those who obliviously puffed away.

The anti-smokers gathered momentum from the lawsuits against, and settlements with, tobacco companies, and they used that leverage to advance their agenda of the systematic eradication of all smoking in anything that could be defined as a public place. Such zealots would love to take that ban to your home and personal property as well, but the Bill of Rights would likely prevail in that battle. Besides, it's easier to just tax smokers into poverty.

Smokers, however, did present an easy target. No one dared to argue the harm and health issues attached to tobacco users as well as those who came into contact with secondhand smoke. The American Cancer Society sponsors several programs designed to promote awareness of the effects of smoking and tools to aid smoking cessation.

Societal pressure currently has smokers on the run and smoking today is clearly on the decline. Just in time, too, as obesity has flexed its, well, whatever it flexes, to supplant smoking as the number one driver of health care costs.

The girth of obesity's wingspan touches a variety of maladies including, but not limited to, hypertension, cholesterol, joint ailments, COPD, cardiovascular, and, the most deadly of them all, diabetes.

It is safe to say that we are in the midst of an obesity epidemic. Pandemic? Bird flu? Unless someone starts deep frying poultry with the bird flu, we're probably safe.

Again, there were no arguments here, Debbie decided. The jury was in, and obesity was the hands down loser in the race to find what was driving the numbers up. Addressing this issue had proven a bit trickier than the smoking issue. That may have been because Americans were, as a nation, both heavier and older than ever. The number of people who were clinically obese represented 31% and many of the rest (65% of the total population) were overweight and headed that direction. This was not a secret. One needed only to fire up the web or visit a local book store to see that among all best sellers were books detailing this diet, that exercise program ad nauseam. There were diet books, diet pills, and diet programs. There were ads, testimonials, gurus, workout videos, you name it.

Debbie recalled her last trip to the grocery store and the number of times she saw the words low fat, lite, no added sugar, fat free, and sugar free. The concept of "heart healthy" had exploded on the scene as if such a label could preclude other poor dietary choices. Debbie chuckled sadly remembering her aunt Polly who, as a diabetic, always ordered a diet Coke to go with the burger and fries. Right.

Still, it was a start. Labels like "low sodium" were helpful to those on low-salt diets to keep hypertension in check. Debbie was still shocked at the fact that over 70% of hypertension was NOT under control with medication.

And there, from the evil of all inactivity, was the fitness channel, as if another reason was necessary to keep inside on the couch. OK, maybe we were getting closer to the problem.

Our schools, pondered Debbie, were now a significant part of the problem as well. The food served by school cafeterias was currently under attack for its poor nutritional content, which was ridiculous when healthy food served with appropriate proportions was cost neutral. Vending machines (hello, not when I went to school, thought Debbie) contained foods inconsistent with a healthy lifestyle, generally with enough sugar to create insulin shock in the healthiest person.

The cruelest blow came in the form of P.E., or Physical Education, in public schools. Debbie thought back to 1985, the year of her graduation from high school. No one ever questioned whether or not to take P.E.; it was understood that everyone participated. Even those who brought the occasional note from the doctor were challenged by teachers and ridiculed by peers into participating at some level.

Today, most schools offered P.E. as an option or required one year to graduate. By default, those who likely needed it the most found other, more sedentary options to involve themselves.

This combination of high-calorie, high-sugar diet and low activity lifestyle was helping to create the next generation of emerging high risk.

All of this, Debbie knew, was deeply ingrained in popular culture and was the result of many years of steady and systematic reinforcement. A change would not be easy or well received.

But Dave, her new benefits consultant, had already burned a core philosophy into her mind: "There is a word in our language for those things that cannot or will not change: *extinct.*" If ever a company was ripe (the definition of ripe included *"almost rotten"*) for a change, it was Goodman Products. "Someone," Debbie thought aloud, "has to be the agent of change, and it doesn't look like there are any other volunteers."

She knew from past experience that she and she alone would be the lightning rod for criticism and derogatory comments, but staying the current course was clearly not an option.

Debbie also was convinced that getting management buy-in, and not just senior management but every level of management, was critical to her success. Clearly, the only difference between a vision and a hallucination was the number of people who saw it.

In her search for wellness strategies, Debbie determined there was no time to ease into a plan over several years; Goodman was at a crossroad and needed relief now. Sometimes it was best to rip the bandage off in one swift, decisive movement.

Debbie's vision for wellness was simple: Those who participated got rewarded, those who chose not to participate were held accountable to financial consequence. Each and every employee would have an equal opportunity to qualify for wellness rewards regardless of his or her current state of health, but it would be a choice, free will. Sort of like the sign in her dentist's office that read, "You don't have to floss all your teeth, just the ones you want to keep."

From time to time, doubts seeped into Debbie's thoughts. "Is this even possible?" was one frequent visitor, although her sense of logic and reason fought back with voluminous, undeniable facts. She had accepted the fact that this would be an uphill climb, literally a cultural reformation. More like a cultural revolution, she mused.

Debbie struggled to suppress her fears of failure, including the phrase she had learned from an organizational development seminar some years back: *Culture eats strategy for lunch, every day!*

The first step in the process recommended by her broker was to develop an aggressive incentive plan. Debbie's wellness plan would include HRAs, or Health Risk Assessments, that she knew would result in some pushback, but were necessary to establish a baseline of current health status. The data collected could also be utilized to offset "worse case" assumptions used by health insurance underwriters absent comprehensive information. The HRA would include family health history, blood pressure, height, weight, and blood draw.

"We're going to lose a few with the blood draw," she thought, "but it's still an employee choice."

The financial incentives required total participation, including the blood draw. It was going to be a showdown.

In addition, each employee would be provided with a device similar to a pedometer called an activity monitor which measured the volume of daily movement and calories burned. Each monitor would be calibrated to reflect the employees height, weight, and age to provide better accuracy.

Periodic challenges and online modules would complement the program and would be accessible via one of many kiosks to be installed specifically for that purpose.

Over time, the goal was simple: the Holy Grail was behavioral change.

The wellness provider recommended by Debbie's broker, Dave, also provided a guaranteed ROI, which reinforced her anticipated success of the program and, more importantly, bridged the gap to the finance department. HR traditionally had always suspected that some form of wellness would bring positive financial results, but until now had faced the wellness conundrum of "It's hard to measure what doesn't happen."

Debbie's broker had also discussed the "Hawthorne effect," the sentinel phenomenon that created behavioral change. "It's most easily described as the way your kids behave when you're watching," Dave explained, "as oppose to when you're not."

Still, the change would be gradual, consistent with most cultural morphs. Debbie prepared herself for the glacial pace, knowing her employees would struggle against change of any kind, but especially in the emotionally charged areas of health care and personal accountability.

She contemplated the members of the leadership team, knowing their complete engagement was the catalyst for success. History reflected well on organizations whose leadership embraced and facilitated change. This was exactly why the final presentation to the team must be compelling and flawless. Without their collective buy in, the risk of failure grew exponentially.

In fact, this whole process of connecting behavior to consequence was little more than "Parenting 101" or training your dog. Yet the degree of difficulty was enormous, for reasons including the fact that employment laws discouraged putting employees in the corner for poor behavioral choices. The use of rolled-up newspapers and shock collars in the workplace was also frowned upon.

Debbie knew that implementing wellness was the right move at the right time; in fact, she was sure of it. And that was important because, deep inside, even with the guaranteed ROI, she knew her career hung in the balance.

YOU HAVE AN UGLY BABY

QUALITY MATTERS

The automakers in Detroit learned this lesson about quality the hard way many years ago: higher quality resulted in lower overall cost. In manufacturing, or any business for that matter, flawed processes, poorly maintained or inappropriately deployed equipment, and human error from lack of training always had the same outcome: higher costs.

Debbie's e-mail notification sounded off and she glanced up to see a meeting invitation from Brenda and her newly recruited benefits team. Both Justin from I.T. and Mike, the director of marketing, would join her and Brenda in their quest for a cultural revolution.

Accepting the meeting scheduled for two PM tomorrow, Debbie forwarded her comments and a draft agenda to the team. Her action items included roll-out meetings, communications strategy, "water cooler" surveys, and buy-in from each departmental manager.

The next morning, Debbie had scarcely logged on when she received an e-mail from John requesting her availability. Although a meeting with John was inevitable, she wanted to put a few more pieces in place before facing the CFO, so she responded with available dates occurring the week after next. John's quick reply revealed concern if not panic, "Is that too late or pushing us too close?"

"We'll be fine," Debbie responded, agreeing to a meeting eleven days out.

After a termination exit interview followed by a grievance and handbook review meeting, Debbie grabbed a quick lunch before meeting with her benefits team.

"Our first order of business," she said, addressing the group, "is to understand that employee benefits here at Goodman are broken. In fact, between the company's cost, employee lack of accountability, and poor quality, I'd say they're downright ugly. But all that is about to change."

"That's what we are already hearing," said Mike. "The guys in the plant are already talking about losing their benefits or paying more for less. And the retirees, they've pretty much accepted the fact that their benefits are history, too."

"Yeah," Justin chimed in. "It's not so bad for the younger guys like me, but it just seems wrong to pull the rug out from under retirees who can least afford it. Especially after working here and helping to build this company."

Fighting the urge to react, Debbie instead focused on being an attentive listener. When Mike and Justin finished, she gathered her thoughts and began. "What we are going to deliver," she started, "is a plan that includes accountability, comprehensive coverage, and quality of care. Our plan will reward positive behavioral change and encourage our co-workers to make smart choices and take better care of themselves and their families."

Debbie continued, "The retirees at Goodman are not going to lose their health care coverage but there will be changes. The free ride is over, but we are not going to abandon the people who helped build this organization. Our new consultant has proposed carving them out into a larger insured pool with the same benefits they have today. Pooling, I have learned, should save us ten to twenty percent today and dramatically impact our long-term FASB liability."

"Sounds like a noble goal," said Mike.

Justin shook his head in disbelief, muttering, "Sounds too good to be true."

Debbie went on. "One of our key initiatives will be 'Quality.' It's not enough that our employees get care, they must get the right care delivered in a high-quality environment, every time."

Brenda wrinkled her nose. "How do we do that? I mean, if you asked our employees by show of hands, nearly all would say their family doctor is above average and we know that can't be true. The fact is the top graduate of Harvard Medical School and the lowest graduate from the worst medical school are called the same thing: Doctor."

Debbie stood up and moved to a white board at the end of the table. On it she wrote: 95% 6 56,000

Turning to her newly recruited team, she queried, "Anyone care to guess what these numbers mean?"

Only Brenda appeared to be thinking, knowing she recognized these numbers from somewhere.

Debbie then let her perplexed teammates off the hook. She said, "Here's what they mean. If ninety-five percent of hospitals performed in six indices like the top five percent, we could avoid 56,000 deaths."

The resulting silence surprised even Debbie. As the words sunk in, Brenda opened her mouth, but nothing came out.

Finally, Justin broke free from his own shock, saying, "I had no idea."

"Even so," muttered Mike, "how do you measure that? Is there a list of underperforming hospitals? And who makes that determination?"

"And what about doctors and other providers?" asked Brenda.

Debbie smiled and said, "Go on, I'm interested in hearing what you are thinking."

"Well," Mike started, raising his eyes to meet Debbie's, "how much will this impact what we're already spending? I mean, you said yourself we had to find ways to reduce costs, so how's that going to balance with all this stuff about higher quality? Don't get me wrong," he backpedaled, "I want higher quality just as much as the next guy, but how are we going to pay for it?"

Summoning her reserves of restraint, Debbie asked, "What about the rest of you, what do you think?"

"I've read about medical mishaps and errors, but I'm at a loss on what to do about it," said Justin. "I just read yesterday that kids get the right medical care about half the time."

Debbie began in a slow, measured response. She explained that in a recent study at Dartmouth University, researchers found that lower quality of care commonly resulted in higher cost, while superior outcomes produced lower overall costs. In fact, using Medicare as a platform which should have generated relatively similar results nationwide, their findings revealed that states spending the lowest average amount produced the highest quality of care. New Hampshire ranked number one in quality and spent the lowest amount per patient, about $5,000. Louisiana, on the other hand, spent the most, over $8,000 per Medicare beneficiary and had the lowest overall quality rating.

"With that in mind—" Debbie began, but was cut off mid-sentence.

Justin couldn't contain his youthful exuberance, blurting out, "So you're saying if we improve the quality of care, cost will go down?"

"Exactly," Debbie confirmed, nodding her head. "Higher quality means getting the appropriate treatment the first time around from the best providers available. That means fewer complications, fewer unnecessary surgeries from incorrect diagnoses, and a lower number of repeated procedures."

"Wow, I would have never thought that in a million years," Mike finally said.

"We'll have help," said Debbie, "from organizations focused on quality health care." "Every employee will have access to HealthGrades™, a great tool for measuring provider outcomes. Our third-party administrator will using filters and standards from The Leapfrog Institute™ and Bridges to Excellence™ to measure frequency, severity, and outcomes of specific procedures. Dave, our new broker, has provided these tools and recommendations to ratchet up our quality awareness.

"It may also be that we choose to remove certain providers from our network based on these findings. I'll need your support when the ensuing noise starts to build."

"Now that you mention it," said Mike sheepishly, "I'm due to have knee surgery in the next six months, and I wouldn't mind knowing which orthopedic surgeon has the best track record for my procedure."

"If you had the tools to check," Debbie asked, "would it matter to you?"

Mike flinched and then said, "You'd be crazy not to!"

"Overall, Americans get the right care about half the time," Debbie added. "The cost of lower quality care is evidenced by repeat office visits, presenteeism, and absenteeism. All of these costs are underwritten by employers with no opportunity for reimbursement." Debbie paused, waiting for comments.

"What else?" asked Justin. He was now engaged, Debbie thought, and his enthusiasm would help drive change the only way it could effectively happen: from the top down.

"Well," Debbie continued, "our prescription provider, called a pharmacy benefit manager, will also have the authority to make clinical edits. Simply put, we are giving them the right to validate what is prescribed based on training and experience. The purpose is to make sure our employees get the right scripts to correspond with the correct diagnosis."

Brenda sighed. "It just never occurred to me to question my providers, prescriptions, or anything."

"We all take a lot for granted, and I'm sure that providers are well meaning." Debbie paused briefly and then added, "You've heard the expression 'To err is human,' but what you have learned is that it is also expensive."

With that, Debbie pushed her chair back and said, "Let's reconvene in a few days. I know this is a lot to download on you at one time. I'm interested in your thoughts after you have had a few days to marinate in the data. I'll send out another meeting invite then."

As Debbie walked down the hall to her office, she reflected on the meeting and her team's responses. "I hope they get it," she pondered, "because they're going to have to defend it."

She knew with certainty that she was moving in the right direction, but still worried about the senior management group. She had learned from observation that the higher you were in an organization, the more toxically joyful you became.

THE FINALE

An exhausted Debbie took a deep breath and held it for a moment. The whirlwind of the last few weeks had finally caught up to her and she felt relief as she exhaled. What had once been a simple exercise of tweaking deductibles and co-pays had evolved into an extensive odyssey into the world of risk management and beyond. With the help and guidance of her new broker, Dave, she had successfully navigated the provider jungle, carefully selecting the best geo access match for her employee population. The networks chosen provided both quality providers and adequate discounts which met Dave and Debbie's standards, as well as several provider options where the company had outlying locations.

With the collective brain trust of her health care committee and input from her benefit consultant, she implemented a program complete with incentives designed to drive participation, but just as importantly signal a change in direction. The message would be clear: Lower cost for those employees who participated in the wellness program, higher cost for those who chose otherwise.

Accountability

The Holy Grail was truly behavioral change. Debbie knew the new direction would not thrill everyone, but failure to disrupt meant absolute failure.

Other pieces were now falling into place. She retained a pharmacy benefit manager recommended by Dave who stressed generics and step therapy. Dave then retained a TPA, not just to adjudicate claims but to screen for fraud, redundancy, and dependent ineligibility.

As part of services provided, Dave, measured and managed the flow of vendors and held to Debbie's timelines and standards. Dave also added a much needed compliance audit covering ERISA, HIPAA, DOL, IRS, as well as handbook and policy/procedure updates.

Although intrigued with the idea of medical travel where procedures done outside the country were much less expensive, Debbie opted to wait until at least next year. Her employees had enough changes to manage with the new focus on wellness. As the savings opportunities continued and credentialing was readily available, medical travel would definitely be a future consideration.

Debbie walked into the main conference room, beaming with a newfound confidence in herself, her decisions, and the new direction for Goodman. Debbie, her benefits team, and her consultant, Dave, had pulled together, with the help of a couple of all-nighters, a masterpiece.

As Debbie took the executive team through her presentation, she watched their eyes grow wide with surprise.

"This year," she said, "is going to be different. For too long we have focused on symptoms and ignored root causes of the rising cost of health insurance. We have methodically shifted costs to our employees through increases in deductibles, co-pays, and employee contributions. In our quest for lower costs we have changed providers, consultants, and plan designs with no appreciable results. In fact, where our benefits are concerned, it's not a pretty picture. If we look at efforts and the results, we have to be truthful enough to admit that *we have an ugly baby.*"

The room went silent with the exception of a few muffled giggles. "Going forward," Debbie continued, "we will focus on the category that contains eighty-two percent of our costs: Claims.

"Our new benefit program will have no changes in coverage, but it will have a restructured contribution strategy. Simply put, employees who participate in the new wellness program will contribute less than those who choose otherwise."

Now eyes were really rolling and brows were raised and wrinkled.

"What about privacy?"

"What about employees who aren't healthy now?"

"We're going to lose key people!"

Dave's insight and forewarning had prepared Debbie for this noise. Debbie straightened and met their concerns headfirst. "Our wellness plan is HIPAA compliant, both privacy and security, which is more than I can say for the rest of our company benefit programs today. The program also meets participants where they are today. For example, if an employee has hypertension, there is no penalty or higher contribution as long as they are on medication and under a doctor's care."

Debbie looked around the table and continued, "I don't want to lose a single employee but, frankly, I fail to see anything negative connected to investing company dollars in the health and well-being of our employees."

The room had almost relaxed until the CEO asked, "How much is this going to cost?"

Debbie smiled and recalled the last meeting with Dave, who also had prepared her for this moment. "It depends," she said, turning to meet his steely gaze. "The cost of implementing wellness for our company is $155,000 per year. The cost of doing nothing," she added, "is a trend increase of thirteen percent on five million dollars. *Guaranteed.*"

Debbie was anxious but anticipated the hush that enveloped the meeting. The CFO had refused to look at her to this moment but glanced up briefly.

"Incidentally, there's a guaranteed ROI, in writing, utilizing Dr. Dee Eddington's methodology for measuring financial efficacy. Bottom line, we implement wellness or get back on this sinking ship."

The CEO stood and Debbie thought, "Oh boy, this is it."

"What do you need from us to make this work?" he asked.

Debbie went for broke. "Well, you have always been an advocate of leading from the top down, so sending the right message means everyone in this room will need to participate."

The CEO went around the table visually and with his hands open asked, "Anyone here have an issue with that?"

And just like that, it was over. This was the biggest moment of her professional career.

With every member of the executive team and every department head engaged, the anticipated pushback was minimal. It turned out that employees were relieved to see benefits unchanged and stepped up to the wellness challenge.

Reviewing the first quarterly claims report, Debbie couldn't help but smile. It was very early, but the jury was in, and the change had produced results: down 11% year over year.

Barely able to contain herself, she e-mailed the report to John, the CFO. "We're on our way!" she typed.

And she remembered the words of Dave, the broker that had guided her through the whole process: "There is a word in our language that defines the inability or unwillingness to change. That word is *extinct*."

THE TEN EMPLOYEE BENEFIT TRUTHS

1. You can't run from your claims (experience).
2. The answer to every insurance question is "It depends."
3. The health care system exists to provide value for its stakeholders, not patients.
4. When you think you have a great strategy involving employee change, remember, "Culture eats strategy for lunch, every day."
5. The only difference between a vision and a hallucination is how many people see it.
6. If your employee benefits strategy doesn't address behavioral change, it's a cost shift.
7. Don't underestimate the power of the "Hawthorne effect."
8. Even if you have a great year financially, you'd better know why.
9. Socialized medicine will not reduce costs, just redistribute costs.
10. To paraphrase Aristotle, "Good health is not an act, but a habit. We are what we repeatedly do."

ABOUT THE AUTHOR

The grandson of a sharecropper and son of a minister, Dan Rickard reflects the homespun wisdom and unshakeable truths with which he was raised.

A licensed insurance agent since 1981, he has provided innovative consulting and brokerage services to both private and publicly held companies, helping to identify and mitigate health-care costs, and works today for a international insurance brokerage firm. He has also served in an advisory capacity and as a board member of numerous insurance companies' agent advisory boards.

Dan lives with his wife, Floellen, and three dogs: Romeo, Juliet, and Heidi.

For speaking engagements and consulting services he can be contacted at dan@youhaveanuglybaby.com

Made in the USA